HENRY WHITWORTH

LIVING WITH

AND

MANAGING

COLON CANCER

BOOK BY: HENRY WHITWORTH

AN EXTENSIVE AID-GIVING SOLUTIONS FOR ADVANCING STOMACH RELATED WELLBEING AND IN GENERAL PROSPERITY

TABLE OF CONTENTS

INTRODUCTION

As we age, the hematopoietic foundational microorganisms that live in the bone marrow and lead to the body's all's unique platelets steadily procure transformations in their DNA. The majority of these changes make no difference, however a can upgrade a specific undifferentiated organism's capacity to get by and multiply, bringing about enormous quantities of platelets that convey a similar transformation, which is known as clonal hematopoiesis.

Clonal hematopoiesis is significantly more every now and again found in patients with numerous different sorts of malignant growth beyond the blood framework and is related with quicker cancer movement and more limited endurance times.

"Be that as it may, whether the presence of clonal hematopoiesis causes the forceful aggregate of irrelevant strong growths has not been energetically tended to."

"Clonal hematopoiesis (CH) is characterized as clonal development of freak hematopoietic undeveloped cells missing determination of a hematologic threat," composed the specialists. "Presence of CH in strong growth patients, including colon disease, associates with more limited endurance. We estimated that bone marrow-determined cells with heterozygous loss-of-capability transformations of DNMT3A, the most widely recognized hereditary modification in CH, add to the pathogenesis of colon malignant growth. In a mouse model that consolidates colitis-related colon malignant growth with exploratory CH driven by Dnmt3a+/Δ, we found higher cancer penetrance and expanded growth trouble contrasted and controls."

The analysts verified that one way clonal hematopoiesis advances the improvement is by expanding the quantity of veins that supply the gastrointestinal cancers with the supplements and oxygen they need to develop.

Hindering the development of these additional veins with axitinib, a medication endorsed by the FDA to treat progressed kidney disease, restrained the development of CAC growths in mice with clonal hematopoiesis.

"Our outcomes show that adjustments in Dnmt3a in bone marrow undifferentiated organisms can significantly affect the advancement through numerous systems, some of which might be restoratively targetable," Guryanova said. "Our discoveries, interestingly, set the causal connection between clonal hematopoiesis and the seriousness of strong cancers and recognize possible helpful systems."

Medical procedure is the main healing methodology for limited colon malignant growth (stage I-III). Careful resection possibly gives the main corrective choice to patients with restricted metastatic sickness in liver or

CHAPTER 1

CRYOTHERAPY

RADIOFREQUENCY REMOVAL

Hepatic blood vessel imbuement of chemotherapeutic specialists

Adjuvant (postoperative) treatment is utilized in chosen patients with stage II colon malignant growth who are at high gamble of repeat, and is standard for stage III colon disease. Regimens utilized for foundational chemotherapy might incorporate the accompanying:

5-Fluorouracil (5-FU)

Capecitabine

Oxaliplatin

Mixes of different specialists (e.g, capecitabine or 5-FU with oxaliplatin, FOLFOX, FOLFIRI, cetuximab or panitumumab with encorafenib)

Regimens utilized for adjuvant chemotherapy generally incorporate 5-FU with leucovorin or capecitabine, either alone or in blend with oxaliplatin.

For metastatic colon malignant growth, fundamental chemotherapy is standard, with neoadjuvant chemotherapy used to change unresectable disengaged liver metastases over completely to resectable liver metastases. Biologic specialists play expected a significant part, normally as designated treatment in view of hereditary examination of the growth. Biologic specialists utilized to treat colon disease incorporate the accompanying:

Obtrusive colorectal malignant growth is a preventable illness. Early location through generally applied screening programs is the main figure the new downfall of colorectal disease in created nations (see Outline/The study of disease transmission).

Major advances in understanding the science and hereditary qualities of colorectal disease are occurring. This information is gradually advancing into the facility and being utilized to all the more likely separate individual dangers of creating colorectal disease, find better screening techniques, consider better visualization, and work on the capacity to foresee benefit from new anticancer treatments.

In the beyond 10 years, an uncommon development in foundational treatment for colorectal malignant growth has emphatically further developed result for patients with metastatic illness. Until the mid-1990s, the main supported specialist for colorectal disease was 5-fluorouracil. From that point forward, new specialists in various classes have opened up, including the accompanying:

Cytotoxic specialists (eg, irinotecan, oxaliplatin)

Oral fluoropyrimidines (ie, capecitabine)

Biologic specialists (e.g, bevacizumab, cetuximab, panitumumab, pembrolizumab, nivolumab)

Most as of late, hostile to angiogenic specialists (ie, ziv-aflibercept, regorafenib)

Despite the fact that medical procedure stays the authoritative therapy methodology, these new specialists will probably convert into further developed fix rates for patients with beginning phase illness (stage II and III) and delayed endurance for those with stage IV sickness. Further advances are probably going to come from the improvement of new designated specialists and from better combination of foundational treatment with different modalities like a medical procedure, radiation treatment, and liver-coordinated treatments.

There are multiple ways of forestalling colon disease. You can lower your risk of developing colon cancer by making changes to your lifestyle, in addition to getting medical tests that aid in the early detection of the disease.

Natural Remedies for Colon Cancer Prevention

Few natural remedies or alternative therapies have been found to be effective in preventing colon cancer to this point. In any case, starter research recommends that the accompanying substances might assist with lessening colon malignant growth chance somewhat. Here is a glance at some key review discoveries:

Vitamin D

High blood levels of vitamin D might be connected to a lower chance of colon malignant growth, as indicated by a recent report. Examining information on 5706 individuals with colorectal malignant growth and 7107 sound people, scientists confirmed that ladies with the most elevated levels of vitamin D had a genuinely huge diminished chance of colon malignant growth contrasted with those with the least levels. For men the gamble was diminished, however not to a measurably critical degree.

Folate

Ensuring you devour sufficient food wellsprings of folate (a B nutrient found in food sources like spinach, asparagus, and sustained grains) may bring down your gamble of colon malignant growth, as per a 2015 orderly survey and meta-examination. Notwithstanding, the examination is blended and more investigations are needed. The suggested day to day admission of folate is 400 micrograms (mcg) for most grown-ups. Women who are breastfeeding should consume 500 mcg per day, while pregnant women should consume 600 mcg per day.

Quercetin

In lab tests on cell societies, researchers have exhibited that quercetin, a cell reinforcement tracked down in tea, may assist with slowing down the development of colon cancer.4 What's more, a 2012 populace based investigation of 2,664 individuals tracked down that dietary admission of quercetin might be connected with decreased chance of colon disease in the proximal colon (first and center parts). Nonetheless, this connection was not found for colon malignant growth in the distal colon (last part) and was not found in the people who previously had a high tea consumption.

Quercetin can be found in foods like apples, onions, and berries naturally as well as in supplements.

Tea According to a 2015 lab study, white tea may protect healthy cells from DNA damage and inhibit the growth of colon cancer cells.

Test-tube and animal-based studies have also shown that green tea can prevent colon cancer. Notwithstanding, the accessible logical information are lacking to reason that any sort of tea might forestall colon disease in people.

Different Ways to deal with Counteraction

To bring down your gamble of colon malignant growth, attempt these procedures suggested by the American Disease Society:

Screening

Evaluating for colorectal disease ought to start at age 45 for all grown-ups at normal gamble, yet at times, prior screening may be fitting. Individuals with a family background of colorectal malignant growth or colon polyps, alongside the people who have incendiary entrails infection ought to talk with their medical care supplier about their gamble and while screening ought to start.

Clinical Rules for Screening

In Spring 2021, the two the U.S. Preventive Administrations Team and the American School of Gastroenterology refreshed their separate clinical rules for colon disease screening to begin at age 45 rather than 50 because of expanding paces of colon malignant growth analyze younger than 50.

Healthy Eating Five or More Servings of a Variety of Fruits and Vegetables a Day, Whole Grains Rather Than Processed Grains, and Reducing Consumption of Red and Processed Meats may Aid in the Prevention of Colon Cancer.

Work out

For colon disease anticipation, hold back nothing 30 minutes of activity on at least five days of the week. Colon cancer risk may be further reduced by engaging in moderate or vigorous activity for at least 45 minutes five or more times per week.

Limiting Alcohol Consumption In addition to quitting smoking, women should drink no more than one drink per day and men should drink no more than two.

Reasons for Colon Disease

As a rule, colon disease starts with the development of precancerous developments (polyps) that become dangerous over the long run. Albeit the reason for colon malignant growth is obscure, the next may build the gamble for the sickness:

Being over 50, having a family history of colon cancer or adenomatous polyps, having a personal history of polyps, having an inherited syndrome linked to colon cancer, not getting enough exercise, eating a diet high in red or processed meat, drinking alcohol, smoking, or being Black Colon Cancer Risk by Race Studies have shown that Black Americans face the highest risk of non-hereditary colon

Black men are even more likely than Black women to die from colorectal cancer. Black women are more likely to die from colorectal cancer than women of any other racial group. The purposes behind these distinctions are hazy.

Symptoms of Colon Cancer although colon cancer typically does not cause symptoms, some patients may experience the following:

Consistent abdominal pain or discomfort Tenderness in the lower abdomen Rectal bleeding or bloody stool Intestinal obstruction Narrow stools

Unexplained weight loss Unexplained anemia Fatigue If you notice any of these symptoms, you should see a doctor right away.

Elective Medication and Colon Malignant growth Avoidance

Because of the absence of science behind their advantages, it's significant not to depend exclusively on any of the above regular cures for of colon malignant growth anticipation. Assuming you're thinking about utilizing regular cures, try to counsel your medical care supplier first. Self-treating and keeping away from or deferring standard consideration can have serious outcomes.

Food sources That Battle Colorectal Disease: A Manual for Nourishment for Counteraction and Treatment

Realize which food sources to eat and stay away from in a colorectal malignant growth therapy diet, as well as the rules for a generally speaking adjusted diet to assist with forestalling colon disease.

Colorectal malignant growth is the third most normal disease analysed in all kinds of people in the U.S., barring skin tumours. While in general paces of individuals being determined to have colorectal malignant growth have diminished every year, youngsters are creating colorectal disease at higher rates than any time in recent memory. In light of this increase, the American

Disease Society brought down the suggested screening age in 2021 from 50 to 45 years of age.

Both treatment and prevention rely heavily on nutrition. The food sources you eat and the way of life you lead influence your malignant growth risk levels and your body's capacity to forestall disease. People who eat well, exercise regularly, keep a healthy weight, and avoid alcohol can reduce their risk of colorectal disease by more than a third, according to some cancer research studies.

Realize what food varieties to pick or lose to accomplish a fair eating regimen for colorectal malignant growth counteraction, in addition to dietary rules to observe during treatment.

What exactly is colon cancer?

Depending on where it begins, colorectal cancer can be referred to as either colon cancer or rectal cancer. Because of their many similar characteristics, these cancers are frequently grouped together.

Risk factors in general, men and women have a lifetime risk of colorectal cancer of approximately one in 23 and one in 26, respectively. Be that as it may, every individual's gamble may be higher or lower contingent upon their gamble factors. Some examples include:

Being overweight or fat

Low active work

Diet

Smoking

Liquor use

Age

Individual or family background of colorectal polyps or colorectal malignant growth

Previous circumstances

Racial or ethnic foundation

The American Malignant growth Society suggests that people at normal gamble start customary screening at 45 years of age.

Day to day dietary decisions for colorectal disease anticipation

The food and beverages you eat can be incredible assets for colorectal disease counteraction. A healthy diet over time can improve your gut health, which is important for the health of your colon and rectal.

Healthy ways to lower your risk of colorectal cancer and prevent it Smart food choices can lower your risk. As a general rule, the American Disease Society suggests that grown-ups and youngsters pick counts calories wealthy in high-fiber food sources, like entire natural products, veggies and entire grains. Rehearses for avoidance include:

Expanding your dietary fiber admission. Eat beans and legumes like pinto beans, black beans, and kidney beans, as well as whole wheat bread and brown rice, which are high in fiber. According to the American Institute for Cancer Research, "Dietary legume consumption reduces the risk of colorectal cancer." These are excellent sources of protein, fiber, vitamin B, and vitamin E.

Consuming a healthy diet. Eat an assortment of plant-based food varieties. Choose whole grains, nuts, beans, vegetables, and other healthy foods. Consume lean protein with some restraint, similar to fish and poultry, and pick low-fat dairy items whenever the situation allows.

Consuming a lot of water. Make sure you get enough fluids every day to stay hydrated. The majority ought to come from drinks that don't contain caffeine.

Dairy consumption. As per the American Establishment for Malignant growth Exploration, there is solid proof that the utilization of dairy can be defensive against colorectal disease.

What to avoid: Consuming certain foods and drinks, particularly in large quantities, can raise your risk of developing colorectal cancer. Reduce your risk by:

Keep away from liquor. Consuming alcohol can make you more likely to get cancerous cells. It transforms into malignant growth causing intensifies in the body, which can likewise harm the cell coating of the colon.

Reevaluate your go-to inexpensive food request. Customarily, cheap food is profoundly handled, low in supplements and may add to heftiness which increments malignant growth risk. Assuming you're when there's no other option and need to snatch lunch in a hurry, attempt a café that utilizes new fixings and offers natural product, vegetables or entire grains as a side dish.

Avoid products that have a lot of glycemic load. Food varieties, for example, white rice, noodles, cake and sugar have a great deal of refined carbs and sugars. You don't need to forego these merchandise out and out however attempt to restrict utilization, as malignant growth research has found an unmistakable and direct connection between food varieties with a high glycemic load and colorectal disease. These increase the likelihood of developing insulin resistance.

Eat less red meat and handled meats. Handled meats and red meats, like store meat or franks, might be related with an expanded gamble of creating colon malignant growth. This is because high-temperature cooking of red meat results in the formation of compounds like polycyclic aromatic hydrocarbons (PAHs) and heterocyclic amines (HCAs). Advanced glycation end products (AGEs), which are substances found in red meat, have also been linked to body inflammation and an increased risk of colorectal cancer.

A brief diet guide: Top food varieties to pick or lose

Stacy Shawhan, enrolled dietitian and affirmed expert in oncology nourishment at the College of Cincinnati Disease Center, realizes how strong eating regimen can be in battling sickness or treating malignant growth. She's a pro at making wholesome designs to help people all through their wellbeing or malignant growth venture.

Stacy offers the following suggestions for avoiding colorectal cancer:

What to pick:

Entire grains. Earthy colored rice, oats, 100 percent entire wheat bread items, quinoa, faro, grain and entire grain pasta.

Dairy items. Cottage cheese, low-fat milk, yogurt, and other cheese products. Malignant growth research proposes the high calcium content in these might be defensive.

Non-boring vegetables and crude natural products. These are high in fiber, which advances stomach wellbeing. These additionally contain phytonutrients known to forestall many sorts of disease.

What to lose:

Alcohol. On the off chance that you really do drink liquor, attempt to do so just incidentally and breaking point to two standard beverages each day for men or one standard beverage each day for ladies

Red and handled meats. Handled meat is any meat (white or dim) that has been safeguarded through salting, smoking or restoring (like salami, wiener, bologna, lunch meats and franks). Both red meat and handled meat contain intensifies that increment the gamble of colon malignant growth.

Stacy's top five colon cancer-fighting foods:

Fish Nutrition for patients undergoing treatment for colorectal cancer when a patient develops colon or rectal cancer, the most common treatments include:

Participation in clinical trials, surgery, chemotherapy, radiation, and a specialized diet can support each treatment type's unique nutritional challenges.

General dietary recommendations for people with colorectal cancer At the University of Cincinnati Cancer Center, we have specialized, oncology-trained dieticians who work with patients to create customized nutrition plans, no matter where they are in their health journey. These plans consider every individual's essential disease therapies and clinical history to advance generally speaking health, results, and patient solace.

Healthful rules for disease treatment

As you move from finding through a medical procedure and different therapies, your dietary requirements will change. When you are receiving treatment for cancer, you should always follow the directions given by your doctor. Changes to your diet, for example, can improve your overall health and help reduce side effects from treatment. Stacy advises you to:

Get sufficient calories. During colorectal cancer treatment, eating enough to keep your weight and muscle mass the same can help patients better tolerate treatment. To keep their weight stable and avoid losing it, many people need more calories after being diagnosed than they did before.

Maintaining a healthy weight is a challenge for many patients. You may not want to eat or drinking during treatment and a few incidental effects could make it hard to eat. But it's important to make sure you get enough calories and fight off unwanted weight loss.

Eat more modest bits. Your body's ability to digest and absorb nutrients is affected by colorectal cancer and its treatment. It is easier for your body to digest food when you eat smaller portions. Try eating smaller portions every two to three hours or adding protein drinks if you have trouble eating large meals.

Incorporate protein with most feasts and bites. Protein is significant for assisting the body with keeping up with muscle and recuperate the harm to solid cells that can be brought about by disease treatment. It can likewise assist your resistant framework with battling contamination and body fix tissues after a medical procedure, chemotherapy or radiation.

Poultry, fish, shellfish, beef, pork, eggs, dairy products like milk, yogurt, cottage cheese, cheese, nuts, nut butter, beans, lentils, and soy products like tofu, edamame, and meat substitutes are all high-protein foods.

Keep hydrated. The essential capability of the colon is to retain water from the food and drinks that we polish off. In the event that you're going through radiation or medical procedure, it very well may be progressively hard for your colon to retain as much water as possible already.

To stay hydrated throughout the day, try drinking water, flavored water, tea, milk, broth, Pedialyte, and sports drinks. Try diluting sugary drinks if you find that they cause you to have loose bowel movements.

Consume sound fats. These give the body energy and decrease irritation, in addition to they might assist the mind and sensory system with working appropriately. They can be found in fish, seeds, nuts, avocados, olive oil, and other foods.

Consult a specialist in nutrition. Malignant growth treatment is exceptionally individualized — as are the nourishment suggestions for every patient's case. Request a referral to a dietitian from your oncologist. A few dietitians work in oncology nourishment — search for dieticians with the letters "RD, CSO," which represents Enrolled Dietitian, Board-Guaranteed Expert in Oncology Sustenance.

Alcohol should be avoided during treatment. It's alright to drink liquor every once in a while, however during treatment, restricting liquor utilization however much as could be expected is significant. Liquor can cooperate with numerous drugs and is connected to the improvement of colon disease. Assuming you do drink, limit your admission to something like one (for ladies) or two (for men) standard drink(s) each day. A typical drink is 12 oz. of beer, 4 oz. of wine, or 1.5 oz. of liquor in a shot.

Herbal and dietary supplements. Supplements are many times considered innocuous. Nonetheless, dietary enhancements (counting nutrients, minerals, herbals and probiotics) can cause adverse consequences during disease treatment. Assuming you're keen on taking dietary enhancements during treatment, make a point to converse with your oncologist or dietician first.

Exploring difficulties and treatment-related aftereffects

While most patients ought to endeavour to follow the overall suggestions for good nourishment during malignant growth treatment, there are times when it's troublesome or not suggested. In certain stages of treatment, side effects such as nausea, diarrhoea, or loss of appetite are common and may necessitate dietary adjustments.

Before making major changes to your diet or way of life, consult your doctor or specialist because your overall health also affects your specific needs.

5 Methods for treating Colon Disease Normally

The advanced medical services foundation would like you to accept that there is just a single genuine method for taking care of any medical problems that you might look in your life. They have strong advertising and campaigning groups, and they strive to safeguard themselves and their strategies. In any case, there really are elective treatments that can be very valuable to the people who are experiencing a portion of this world's most difficult diseases. For instance, there are natural and alternative treatments for colon cancer that can help you fight the disease naturally. Can colon cancer be treated naturally? Is there an option in contrast to chemotherapy or radiation? Today, we'll look at the various natural ways to get rid of colon cancer.

Like different kinds of malignant growth, colon disease is analyzed in stages, and thorough treatment is many times subject to what point the sickness is analyzed.

Colon Malignant growth | Stage

While examining colon disease arranges, a few patients are shocked to catch wind of Stage 0. Polyps of cancer cells only found in the inner lining (or mucosa) of the colon or rectum are referred to as cancer in situ at this stage. These harmful cells in colon polyps can be eliminated during a polypectomy, part of a colonoscopy.

Colon Disease | Stage I

Stage I of colon disease is malignant growth that has outgrown the inward covering and into the layers of muscle on the colon or rectum. However, it has not yet reached other lymph nodes or tissues.

Colon Disease | Stage II

Stage II happens when the disease has spread past the colon wall however not into the lymph hubs. This stage is isolated into three distinct areas.

Stage IIA

In this stage, the malignant growth has spread through the walls however not to the lymph hubs.

Stage IIB

Stage IIB implies the malignant growth has spread through the instinctive peritoneum, the layers of muscle covering the mid-region. It hasn't spread elsewhere or to the lymph hubs.

Stage IIC

In this stage, the cancer has developed through the wall and spread to local designs. It has not reached the lymph nodes or anywhere else.

Stage III of Colon Cancer: When cancer has spread beyond the lining of the colon to the lymph nodes, it is considered stage III. Albeit the malignant growth influences the lymph hubs at this stage, it hasn't spread to different organs inside the body. This stage, like stage II before it, is broken down into three distinct categories.

Stage IIIA

Here, the malignant growth has developed through the muscle layers of the digestive tract and has spread to 1-3 lymph hubs (or to a knob of cancer in the tissues encompassing the colon or rectum that don't seem like lymph hubs) yet has not spread somewhere else.

Stage IIIB: The cancer has either spread through the wall or to surrounding organs and 1-3 lymph nodes (or to a nodule of tumor in the tissues surrounding the colon or rectum that does not appear to be a lymph node), but it has not spread to other parts of the body in Stage IIIB.

Stage IIIC

The malignant growth has spread to at least four lymph hubs in this stage. It hasn't spread to other far off region of the body.

Colon Cancer | Stage IV When colon cancer reaches stage IV, it has spread to other organs in the body through the blood and lymph nodes. This stage can be separated into three distinct classifications too.

Stage IVA

Colon disease has spread to one single far off piece of the body (like the lungs or liver).

Colon cancer of stage IVB has spread to multiple organs.

Colon or rectal cancer in stage IVC has spread to the peritoneum, which is the membrane that linings the abdominal cavity, and may have spread to other organs or sites.

Colon cancer can be treated, depending on the stage and affected areas.

1. Create a Healthy Diet The majority of people are aware that they should eat better to improve their lives. In any case, many don't understand that eating better could help colon disease treatment. We as a whole should eat specific food varieties and drinks, and there are others we should stay away from. For instance, the foods that fight cancer and are high in omega-3 fatty acids should be consumed:

Salmon

Halibut

Entire grains

Verdant green vegetables

These are the sort of things that can reinforce your invulnerable framework and make it more straightforward for that framework to retaliate against the issues that are frequently connected with colon disease.

In addition to focusing on what you should be eating, it is ideal for avoiding other foods and beverages that could impede your progress. A large number of the food varieties and refreshments that fall into this classification are the standard suspects. You should steer clear of, for instance:

Foods with a lot of fat or that have been fried Red meat Alcohol At the very least, it is recommended that you limit your intake of these foods and drinks. The majority of people find it difficult to completely avoid these substances, but even consuming them in moderation can be extremely beneficial to your body's ability to fight off illness and disease.

Natural treatment for colon cancer. Find out more!

2. Investigate Botanical Treatments Numerous cancer specialists and other members of the healthcare industry are ecstatic over the findings of recent studies that suggest that the use of botanical treatments in conjunction with other treatments may aid in the fight against colon cancer.

The regular organic known as Andrographis paniculata is what the absolute most recent examinations have focused in on. Malignant growth research shows that Andrographis paniculata might be valuable in aiding battle colon disease that has been impervious to chemotherapy.

The objective of the study was to find a natural substance that would not only be nontoxic when exposed to chemotherapy but could also aid in the treatment of colon cancer. The analysts realize that a great many people with colon malignant growth would probably have gotten chemotherapy eventually during their determination or would get chemotherapy sooner or later. As a result, they needed to locate something that would not interact adversely with chemotherapy. Luckily, apparently Andrographis paniculata fits that bill.

What functions Andrographis Paniculata?

This organic is basically tracked down in South Asia, yet it can likewise be tracked down in the US. It is as of now referred to for its mitigating properties as well concerning being antibacterial and antiviral. It has recently received even more attention because of its potential to fight colon cancer cells.

It is expressed that it wasn't surprising to analysts that Andrographis killed malignant growth cells. There was at that point adequate proof that it could do this even before his review grabbed hold. What was more fascinating was the capacity of Andrographis to kill purported malignant growth "supercells." These colon malignant growth cells have shown to be impervious to chemotherapy and other normal disease medicines.

Scientists chipped away at creature examples first to guarantee their tests would function true to form. They then moved on to a 3D-organoid model made from human colorectal tumor tissue taken from a real cancer patient after getting encouraging results there. By and by, the test demonstrated that the utilization of Andrographis worked on the utilization of chemotherapy without help from anyone else. It appears to be that Andrographis, in blend with chemotherapy and other suggested medicines, perhaps the response that specialists have been searching for.

3. Green tea has been shown to reduce the risk of colon cancer in both men and women in studies. Strangely, this is what is going on in which the examinations have created a few clashing information. In one review, the information show that ladies who drink at least 5 cups of green tea everyday see a few advantages in colon malignant growth counteraction and improvement. In any case, a similar impact was not tracked down in men. Extra examinations have likewise proposed that tea utilization overall (counting non-green tea) is valuable in colon malignant growth anticipation in ladies. By and by, a similar exploration has not shown valuable effects for tycoons to forestall colon disease.

CHAPTER 2

Pathophysiology

Hereditarily, colorectal malignant growth addresses a complicated illness, and hereditary changes are frequently connected with movement from premalignant injury (adenoma) to intrusive adenocarcinoma. Grouping of atomic and hereditary occasions prompting change from adenomatous polyps to unmistakable threat has been portrayed by Vogelstein and Fearon. [6]

The early occasion is a transformation of APC (adenomatous polyposis quality), which was first found in quite a while with familial adenomatous polyposis (FAP). The protein encoded by APC is significant in the actuation of oncogene c-myc and cycling D1, which drives the movement to threatening aggregate. Despite the fact that FAP is an uncommon genetic disorder representing just around 1% of instances of colon disease, APC transformations are extremely regular in irregular colorectal tumours.

Other significant qualities in colon carcinogenesis incorporate the KRAS oncogene, chromosome 18 loss of heterozygosis (LOH) prompting inactivation of SMAD4 (DPC4), and DCC (erased in colon malignant growth) cancer concealment qualities. Chromosome arm 17p erasure and transformations influencing the p53 growth silencer quality present protection from customized cell deat — h (apoptosis) and are believed to be late occasions in colon carcinogenesis.

A subset of colorectal malignant growths is described with lacking DNA confuse fix. This aggregate has been connected to transformations of qualities like MSH2, MLH1, and PMS2. These transformations result in purported high recurrence microsatellite unsteadiness (H-MSI), which can be distinguished with an immunocytochemistry examine. H-MSI is a sign of genetic nonpolyposis colon disease disorder (HNPCC, Lynch condition), which represents around 6% of all colon malignant growths. H-MSI is additionally viewed as in around 20% of irregular colon diseases.

Notwithstanding transformations, epigenetic occasions, for example, strange DNA methylation can likewise cause quieting of growth silencer qualities or actuation of oncogenes. These occasions compromise the hereditary equilibrium and at last lead to harmful change.

Disease cells produce extracellular vesicles (EVs) — basically, microvesicles and exosomes — that can advance the development, endurance, obtrusiveness, and metastatic action of growths. [7] Zhao et al detailed that in a creature model of forceful late-stage colorectal malignant growth, cancer emitted EVs elevated protection from safe designated spot barricade. The colorectal disease cells in this model emit exosomes that convey immunosuppressive microRNAs these block CD28 on Lymphocytes and CD80 on dendritic cells that penetrate the cancers, impairing Lymphocyte intervened enemy of growth resistant reaction.

Further, these creators found that intravenous infusions of cancer discharged exosomes without immunosuppressive microRNAs, in blend with resistant designated spot inhibitors, brought about an improved enemy of growth safe reaction. This offers a likely restorative technique for late-stage colorectal disease.

Etiology

Colorectal malignant growth is a multifactorial sickness process. Hereditary elements, natural openings (counting diet), and fiery states of gastrointestinal system are undeniably associated with the advancement of colorectal malignant growth.

Albeit much about colorectal malignant growth hereditary qualities stays obscure, flow research demonstrates that hereditary variables have the best connection to colorectal disease. Genetic change of the APC quality is the reason for familial adenomatous polyposis (FAP), in which impacted people convey a practically 100 percent hazard of creating colon malignant growth by age 40 years.

Inherited nonpolyposis colon disease disorder (HNPCC, Lynch condition) presents about a 40% lifetime risk for creating colorectal malignant growth; people with this condition are likewise at expanded risk for urothelial malignant growth, endometrial malignant growth, and other more uncommon tumors. Lynch condition is described by lacking bungle fix (dMMR) because of acquired change in one of the confound fix qualities, like hMLH1, hMSH2, hMSH6, hPMS1, hPMS2, and possibly not discover other genes.

HNPCC is a reason for around 6% of all colon malignant growths. Albeit the utilization of ibuprofen might decrease the gamble of colorectal neoplasia in certain populaces, a concentrate by Consume et al tracked down no impact on the occurrence of colorectal malignant growth in transporters of Lynch condition with utilization of headache medicine, safe starch, or both.

Dietary variables are the subject of extraordinary and progressing examinations. Epidemiologic examinations have connected expanded chance of colorectal malignant growth with an eating routine high in red meat and creature fat, low-fiber diets, and low generally admission of leafy foods. A concentrate by Aune et al observed that a high admission of fiber was related with a decreased gamble of colorectal disease. Specifically, cereal fiber and entire grains were viewed as successful. A concentrate by Pala et al observed that high yogurt admission was likewise connected with a diminished gamble for colorectal malignant growth.

Heftiness and way of life decisions, for example, cigarette smoking, liquor utilization, and stationary propensities have likewise been related with expanded risk for colorectal malignant growth. A meta-examination of planned companion concentrates on found a humble yet huge height of colorectal disease risk in momentum smokers; risk was higher for men and for rectal tumors than colon malignant growths, and enduring in previous smokers.

In an enormous imminent review, Cho and partners revealed that high liquor utilization was related with raised risk for colorectal malignant growth, in people with a family background of the sickness. The affiliation was huge just for the most elevated liquor admission class of 30 g or all the more day to day; no critical straight pattern was apparent. In examination with nondrinkers with no family ancestry, people who polished off 30 g/d or more and who had a family background of colorectal malignant growth had a relative gamble for colon malignant growth of 2.80.

Current screening rules suggest that clinicians know about expanded colorectal disease risk in patients who smoke or are corpulent, however don't feature the expanded gamble in patients with diabetes. A meta-examination of case-control and partner concentrates on recognized diabetes as a free gamble factor for colon and rectal malignant growth. Subgroup investigations affirmed the consistency of the discoveries across concentrate on type and populace. This data might affect screening rules and on building risk models of colorectal malignant growth.

Age is a notable gamble factor for colorectal malignant growth, all things considered for the vast majority other strong cancers. The course of events for movement from early premalignant injury to harmful malignant growth goes from 10-20 years. Middle age at conclusion is 66 years.

Be that as it may, rather than the decrease in colon disease occurrence rates in people age 55 and more seasoned, which started during the 1980s, paces of colon malignant growth in more youthful people have been expanding. In grown-ups age 20 to 39 years, colon disease occurrence rates have expanded by 1.0% to 2.4% yearly since the mid-1980s; in those age 40 to 54 years, the frequency has expanded by 0.5% to 1.3% every year since the mid-1990s. At present, grown-ups conceived around 1990 have twofold the gamble of colon disease contrasted and those conceived around 1950. Expanded heftiness is one probably factor.

From 2011 through 2016, the frequency of colorectal malignant growth kept on declining in those matured 65 years and more established, by 3.3% every year. Rates expanded by 1% yearly in those matured 50 to 64 years, and rose around 2% every year in those more youthful than 50 years. The American Malignant growth Society assessed that 17,930 of the 147,950 people expected to be determined to have colon and rectal disease in 2020, and 3640 of the 53,200 expected to kick the bucket from the illness, would be more youthful than 50 years old.

Growth site will in general change by persistent age. From 2012 to 2016, the proximal colon was the site of colon malignant growth in 23% of those under 50 years old, 31% of those 50-64 years, and 49% of those 65 and more established. Occurrence patterns fluctuated by race/identity: in those 50-64 years of age, rates expanded in whites by 1.3% each year however diminished in blacks by 1.6% each year, and were steady in Hispanics. In those more youthful than 50, rates increased by 2% every year in whites and by 0.5% yearly in Blacks.

Visualization

The surmised 5-year endurance rate for colorectal malignant growth patients in the (every one of us stages included) is 64.6%. [23] Endurance is conversely connected with stage: inexact 5-year relative endurance rates are as per the following:

Restricted infection: 90.2%

Territorial infection: 71.8%

Far off illness: 14.3%

A concentrate by Chua et al found that roughly one in each three patients who go through resection for colorectal liver metastases become genuine 5-year survivors. [32] Of those, roughly half endure 10 years and are relieved of colorectal liver metastases. A multivariate investigation of 1001 patients who went through possibly corrective resection of liver metastases recognized five elements as free indicators of more terrible result.

Size more noteworthy than 5 cm

Infection free time period than a year

More than one cancer

Essential lymph-hub inspiration

Carcinoembryonic antigen (CEA) level more noteworthy than 200 ng/mL

Aggarwal et al found that flowing growth cells estimated at standard after the commencement of new treatment in patients with metastatic colorectal disease freely anticipated endurance; in patients with a gauge carcinoembryonic antigen (CEA) worth of 25 ng/mL or higher, those with low benchmark levels of coursing cancer cells (< 3) had longer endurance. Both the quantity of coursing growth cells and the CEA level estimated at 6-12 weeks freely anticipated endurance.

Research proposes a job for intra-tumoral resistant reaction as an indicator of clinical result in patients with colorectal disease, notwithstanding more conventional obsessive and sub-atomic markers. Katz et al revealed that in patients with colorectal liver metastases, big quantities of T administrative cells comparative with CD4 or CD8 Lymphocytes anticipated unfortunate result

The standard utilization of adjunctive specialists for inside purging before colonoscopy (eg, simethicone, enhanced electrolyte arrangements, prokinetics, spasmolytic, bisacodyl, senna, olive oil, and probiotics is) isn't suggested. Be that as it may, extra entrail laxatives ought to be viewed as in patients with risk factors for deficient readiness (eg, patients with an earlier lacking planning, history of obstruction, utilization of narcotics or other clogging prescriptions, earlier colon resection, diabetes mellitus, or spinal rope injury).

In spite of the fact that sodium phosphate (Rest) is viable and very much endured by most patients, the gamble of unfavourable occasions makes it unsatisfactory as a first-line specialist. Rest ought to be stayed away from in old patients and in patients with known or thought fiery entrail illness.

Low-volume arrangements or expanded time conveyance for high-volume arrangements are suggested for patients after bariatric medical procedure.

For screening, patients with one first-degree relative determined to have colorectal malignant growth or high level adenoma at age 60 years or more established are considered at normal gamble. For patients with a solitary first-degree relative determined to have colorectal malignant growth or high level adenoma before age 60 years, or those with two first-degree family members with colorectal disease or high level adenomas, the rule suggests colonoscopy like clockwork, starting at age 40 years or at 10 years more youthful than the age at finding of the most youthful impacted family member.

Being determined to have colon malignant growth can achieve various sentiments. Why me? What are my treatment choices? What will the aftereffects be like? Could I at any point deal with myself? Will this effect how long I live?

A conclusion of stage II colon malignant growth has an additional worry do I want chemotherapy after medical procedure? The response is, "Perhaps." Studies have not tracked down an unambiguous response to this inquiry as a rule. Chemotherapy makes side impacts and we would rather not superfluously open individuals to chemotherapy except if we are sure aiding them is going.

Therapies utilized for colorectal malignant growth might incorporate a mix of a medical procedure, radiation treatment, chemotherapy, and focused on therapy.[5] Tumors that are limited to the mass of the colon might be reparable with medical procedure, while disease that has spread generally is normally not treatable, with the executives being coordinated towards working on personal satisfaction and symptoms.[5] The five-year endurance rate in the US was around 65% in 2014.[6] The singular probability of endurance really relies on how cutting-edge the disease is, whether all the malignant growth can be taken out with a medical procedure, and the individual's by and large health.[1] Worldwide, colorectal disease is the third most normal sort of disease, making up around 10% of all cases.[14] In 2018, there were 1.09 million new cases and 551,000 passings from the disease.[8] It is more considered normal in created nations, where over 65% of cases are found.[2] It is less considered normal in ladies than men.[2]

Signs and side effects

The signs and side effects of colorectal malignant growth rely upon the area of the cancer in the entrail, and whether it has spread somewhere else in the body (metastasis). The exemplary admonition signs include: demolishing clogging, blood in the stool, decline in stool type (thickness), loss of hunger, deficiency of weight, and sickness or heaving in somebody north of 50 years old. Around half of individuals who have colorectal malignant growth don't report any symptoms.

Cause

75-95% of colorectal disease cases happen in individuals with next to zero hereditary risk.[19][20] Hazard factors incorporate more seasoned age, male sex,[20] high admission of fat, sugar, liquor, red meat, handled meats, corpulence, smoking, and an absence of physical exercise.[19][21] The Rectal Malignant growth Endurance Mini-computer created by the MD Anderson Malignant growth Place furthermore believes competition to be a gamble factor; notwithstanding, there are value issues concerning whether this could prompt disparity in clinical choice making.[22][23] Roughly 10% of cases are connected to deficient activity.[24] The gamble from liquor seems to increment at more noteworthy than one beverage for each day.[25] Drinking five glasses of water a day is connected to a lessening in the gamble of colorectal disease and adenomatous polyps.[26] Streptococcus gallolyticus is related with colorectal cancer.[27] A few types of Streptococcus bovis/Streptococcus equinus complex are polished off by a large number of individuals day to day and hence might be safe.[28] 25 to 80% of individuals with Streptococcus bovis/gallolyticus bacteremia have corresponding colorectal tumors.[29] Seroprevalence of Streptococcus bovis/gallolyticus is considered as a competitor down to earth marker for the early expectation of a basic entrail sore at high gamble population.[29] It has been recommended that the presence of antibodies to Streptococcus bovis/gallolyticus antigens or the actual antigens in the circulation system might go about as markers for the carcinogenesis in the colon.[29]

Individuals with fiery entrail illness (ulcerative colitis and Crohn's sickness) are at expanded hazard of colon cancer.[31][32] The gamble builds the more drawn out an individual has the infection, and the more regrettable the seriousness of inflammation.[33] In these high gamble gatherings, both counteraction with ibuprofen and normal colonoscopies are recommended.[34] Endoscopic observation in this high-risk populace might decrease the improvement of colorectal malignant growth through early conclusion and may likewise diminish the possibilities passing.

HENRY WHITWORTH

CHAPTER 3

HEREDITARY QUALITIES

Those with a family ancestry in at least two first-degree family members (like a parent or kin) have a two to triple more serious gamble of sickness, and this gathering represents around 20% of all cases. Various hereditary disorders are likewise connected with higher paces of colorectal disease. The most widely recognized of these is genetic nonpolyposis colorectal disease (HNPCC, or Lynch condition) which is available in around 3% of individuals with colorectal cancer.[20] Different disorders that are unequivocally connected with colorectal malignant growth incorporate Gardner condition and familial adenomatous polyposis (FAP).[35] For individuals with these disorders, malignant growth quite often happens and makes up 1% of the disease cases.[36] A complete proctocolectomy might be suggested for individuals with FAP as a preventive measure because of the great gamble of danger. Colectomy, evacuation of the colon, may not get the job done as a preventive measure in view of the great gamble of rectal disease if the rectum remains.[37] The most well-known polyposis disorder influencing the colon is serrated polyposis syndrome,[38] which is related with a 25-40% gamble of CRC.

Most passing because of colon malignant growth are related with metastatic infection. A quality that seems to add to the potential for metastatic sickness, metastasis related in colon disease 1 (MACC1), has been isolated.[41] It is a transcriptional factor that impacts the outflow of hepatocyte development factor. This quality is related with the multiplication, attack, and dissipating of colon disease cells in cell culture, and cancer development and metastasis in mice. MACC1 might be an expected objective for malignant growth mediation, yet this chance should be affirmed with clinical studies.[42]

Epigenetic factors, for example, strange DNA methylation of growth silencer advertisers, assume a part in the improvement of colorectal cancer.[43]

Ashkenazi Jews have a 6% higher gamble pace of getting adenomas and afterward colon malignant growth because of changes in the APC quality being more common.[44]

Pathogenetics

Colorectal malignant growth is an illness beginning from the epithelial cells covering the colon or rectum of the gastrointestinal plot, most often because of hereditary changes in the Wnt flagging pathway that increments flagging activity.[45] The Wnt flagging pathway typically assumes a significant part for ordinary capability of these phones including keeping up with this coating. Transformations can be acquired or procured, and most presumably happen in the digestive tomb stem cell.[46][47][48] The most usually changed quality in all colorectal malignant growth is the APC quality, which creates the APC protein.[45] The APC protein forestalls the collection of β-catenin protein. Without APC, β-catenin aggregates to significant levels and moves (moves) into the core, ties to DNA, and enacts the record of proto-oncogenes. These qualities are regularly significant for undeveloped cell restoration and separation, yet when improperly communicated at undeniable levels, they can cause cancer.[45] While APC is changed in most colon tumors, a few malignant growths have expanded β-catenin due to transformations in β-catenin (CTNNB1) that block its own breakdown, or have transformations in different qualities with capability like APC like AXIN1, AXIN2, TCF7L2, or NKD1.

Past the deformities in the flagging pathway, different changes should happen for the cell to become harmful. The p53 protein, delivered by the TP53 quality, ordinarily screens cell division and actuates their modified passing in the event that they have Wnt pathway deserts. In the long run, a cell line gets a change in the TP53 quality and changes the tissue from a harmless epithelial growth into an obtrusive epithelial cell disease. In some cases the quality encoding p53 isn't changed, however another defensive protein named BAX is transformed instead.

Different proteins answerable for customized cell passing that are generally deactivated in colorectal diseases are TGF-β and DCC (Erased in Colorectal Malignant growth). TGF-β has a deactivating change in portion of colorectal malignant growths. In some cases TGF-β isn't deactivated, however a downstream protein named SMAD is deactivated.[49] DCC usually has an erased portion of a chromosome in colorectal cancer.[50]

Roughly 70% of all human qualities are communicated in colorectal malignant growth, with simply more than 1% of having expanded articulation in colorectal disease contrasted with different types of cancer.[51] A few qualities are oncogenes: they are overexpressed in colorectal disease. For instance, qualities encoding the proteins KRAS, RAF, and PI3K, which ordinarily animate the cell to partition because of development factors, can obtain transformations that outcome in over-enactment of cell expansion. The sequential request of changes is now and again significant. On the off chance that a past APC change happened, an essential KRAS transformation frequently advances to malignant growth as opposed to a self-restricting hyperplastic or fringe lesion.[52] PTEN, a growth silencer, regularly restrains PI3K, yet can some of the time become changed and deactivated.[49]

Far reaching, genome-scale examination has uncovered that colorectal carcinomas can be sorted into hypermutated and non-hypermutated growth types.[53] notwithstanding the oncogenic and inactivating transformations depicted for the qualities above, non-hypermutated tests additionally contain changed CTNNB1, FAM123B, SOX9, ATM, and ARID1A. Advancing through an unmistakable arrangement of hereditary occasions, hypermutated growths show changed types of ACVR2A, TGFBR2, MSH3, MSH6, SLC9A9, TCF7L2, and BRAF. The normal topic among these qualities, across both growth types, is their contribution in Want and TGF-β flagging pathways, which brings about expanded movement of MYC, a key participant in colorectal cancer.[53]

Jumble fix (MMR) lacking growths are portrayed by a somewhat high measure of poly-nucleotide couple repeats.[54] This is brought about by a lack in MMR proteins - which are regularly brought about by epigenetic quieting or potentially acquired changes (e.g., Lynch syndrome).[55] 15 to

18 percent of colorectal disease growths have MMR inadequacies, with 3% creating due to Lynch syndrome.[56] The job of the befuddle fix framework is to safeguard the uprightness of the hereditary material inside cells (i.e., blunder identifying and correcting).[55] Subsequently, a lack in MMR proteins might prompt a failure to distinguish and fix hereditary harm, considering further malignant growth making transformations happen and colorectal disease to progress.[55]

The polyp to malignant growth movement succession is the old style model of colorectal disease pathogenesis.[57] In this adenoma-carcinoma grouping, [58] ordinary epithelial cells progress to dysplastic cells like adenomas, and afterward to carcinoma, by a course of moderate hereditary mutation.[59] Fundamental to the polyp to CRC arrangement are quality transformations, epigenetic modifications, and neighborhood fiery changes.[57] The polyp to CRC succession can be utilized as a hidden structure to show how explicit sub-atomic changes lead to different malignant growth subtypes.

Epigenetics

Epigenetic modifications are significantly more successive in colon disease than hereditary (mutational) changes. As depicted by Vogelstein et al.,[66] a typical disease of the colon has just 1 or 2 oncogene transformations and 1 to 5 cancer silencer changes (together assigned "driver changes"), with around 60 further "traveller" transformations. The oncogenes and growth silencer qualities are all around contemplated and are depicted above under Pathogenesis.

Notwithstanding epigenetic adjustment of articulation of miRNAs, other normal sorts of epigenetic modifications in malignant growths that change quality articulation levels incorporate direct hyper methylation or hypomethylation of CpG islands of protein-encoding qualities and changes in histones and chromosomal engineering that impact quality expression.[71] for instance, 147 hypermethylations and 27 hypomethylations of protein coding qualities were much of the time related with colorectal tumors. Of the hypermethylated qualities, 10 were hypermethylated in 100 percent of colon diseases, and numerous others were hypermethylated in over half of colon cancers.[72] likewise, 11 hypermethylations and 96 hypomethylations of miRNAs were likewise connected with colorectal cancers.[72] Strange (deviant) methylation happens as an ordinary result of typical maturing and the gamble of colorectal malignant growth increments as an individual gets older.[73] The source and trigger of this age-related methylation is unknown.[73][74] Roughly 50% of the qualities that show age-related methylation changes are the very qualities that have been recognized to be engaged with the improvement of colorectal cancer.[73] These discoveries might propose a justification for age being related with the expanded gamble of creating colorectal cancer.

Epigenetic decreases of DNA fix catalyst articulation may probably prompt the genomic and epigenomic unsteadiness normal for cancer.[75][76][67] As summed up in the articles Carcinogenesis and Neoplasm, for irregular malignant growths by and large, a lack in DNA fix is once in a while because of a transformation in a DNA fix quality, however is substantially more regularly due to epigenetic modifications that diminish or quietness articulation of DNA fix genes.

Epigenetic modifications engaged with the improvement of colorectal malignant growth might influence an individual's reaction to chemotherapy.[78]

Genomics and Epigenomics

Agreement sub-atomic subtypes (CMS) order of colorectal malignant growth was first presented in 2015. CMS order up until this point has been viewed as the most powerful grouping framework that anyone could hope to find for CRC that has a reasonable organic interpretability and the reason for future clinical delineation and subtype-based designated interventions.[79]

A clever Epigenome-based Order (EpiC) of colorectal malignant growth was proposed in 2021 presenting 4 enhancer subtypes in individuals with CRC. Chromatin states utilizing 6 histone marks are portrayed to distinguish EpiC subtypes. A combinatorial remedial methodology in light of the recently presented agreement sub-atomic subtypes (CMSs) and Stories could fundamentally improve current treatment strategies.[80]

Conclusion

Colon malignant growth with broad metastases to the liver

Colorectal malignant growth determination is performed by testing of region of the colon dubious for conceivable cancer improvement, regularly during colonoscopy or sigmoidoscopy, contingent upon the area of the lesion.[20] It is affirmed by microscopical assessment of a tissue test.

Presence of not entirely set in stone by a CT sweep of the chest, midsection and pelvis.[20] Other potential imaging tests, for example, PET and X-ray might be utilized in certain cases.[20] X-ray is especially helpful to decide neighbourhood phase of the cancer and to design the ideal careful approach.[81]

X-ray is additionally performed after culmination of neoadjuvant chemoradiotherapy to distinguish patients who accomplish total reaction. Patients with complete reaction on both X-ray and endoscopy may not need careful resection and can keep away from superfluous careful bleakness and complications.[82] Patients chose for non-careful therapy of rectal disease ought to have occasional X-ray checks, get actual assessments, and go through endoscopy methods to identify any growth re-development which can happen in a minority of these patients. At the point when nearby repeat happens, occasional follow up can identify it when it is still little and treatable with rescue a medical procedure. Likewise, X-ray growth relapse grades can be allotted after chemoradiotherapy which relate with patients' drawn out endurance outcomes.

Arranging

Primary article: Colon malignant growth organizing

Arranging of the malignant growth depends on both radiological and neurotic discoveries. Likewise with most different types of malignant growth, cancer organizing depends on the TNM framework which thinks about how much the underlying growth has spread and the presence of metastases in lymph hubs and more far off organs.[20] The AJCC eighth version was distributed in 2018.[89]

Avoidance

It has been assessed that about portion of colorectal disease cases are because of way of life factors, and about a fourth of all cases are preventable.[90] Expanding reconnaissance, participating in active work, polishing off an eating routine high in fiber, and diminishing smoking and liquor utilization decline the risk.[91][92]

Way of life

Way of life risk factors major areas of strength for with incorporate absence of activity, cigarette smoking, liquor, and obesity.[93][94][95] The gamble of colon malignant growth can be decreased by keeping an ordinary body weight through a mix of adequate activity and eating a sound diet.[96]

Flow research reliably connects eating more red meat and handled meat to a higher gamble of the disease.[97] Beginning during the 1970s, dietary proposals to forestall colorectal malignant growth frequently included expanding the utilization of entire grains, leafy foods, and diminishing the admission of red meat and handled meats. This depended on creature studies and review observational examinations. In any case, huge scope imminent examinations have neglected to show a critical defensive impact, and because of the various reasons for malignant growth and the intricacy of concentrating on connections among's diet and wellbeing, it is dubious whether a particular dietary mediations will have critical defensive effects.[98]: 432-433 [99]: 125-126 Of every 2018 the Public Disease

Foundation expressed that "There is no solid proof that an eating routine began in adulthood that is low in fat and meat and high in fiber, organic products, and vegetables lessens the gamble of CRC by a clinically significant degree."[93][100]

As indicated by the World Malignant growth Exploration Asset, polishing off cocktails and consuming handled meat both increment the gamble of colorectal disease.

Higher actual work is recommended.[21][105] Actual activity is related with an unobtrusive decrease in colon yet not rectal malignant growth risk.[106][107] Elevated degrees of actual work lessen the gamble of colon disease by around 21%.[108] Sitting consistently for delayed periods is related with higher mortality from colon malignant growth. Ordinary activity doesn't discredit the gamble however brings down it.

Drug and enhancements

Headache medicine and celecoxib seem to diminish the gamble of colorectal malignant growth in those at high risk Ibuprofen is prescribed in the people who are 50 to 60 years of age, don't have an expanded gamble of dying, and are in danger for cardiovascular sickness to forestall colorectal cancer. It isn't suggested in those at normal risk.

Screening

As over 80% of colorectal tumors emerge from adenomatous polyps, evaluating for this disease is successful for both early recognition and for prevention. Determination of instances of colorectal malignant growth through screening will in general happen 2-3 years before analysis of cases with symptoms.[20] Any polyps that are identified can be eliminated, normally by colonoscopy or sigmoidoscopy, and consequently keep them from transforming into disease. Screening can possibly diminish colorectal malignant growth passing by 60%.[118]

The three principal screening tests are colonoscopy, waste mysterious blood testing, and adaptable sigmoidoscopy. Of the three, no one but sigmoidoscopy can't screen the right half of the colon where 42% of tumors are found.[119] Adaptable sigmoidoscopy, in any case, has the best proof for diminishing the gamble of death from any cause.

Waste mysterious blood testing (FOBT) of the stool is commonly suggested like clockwork and can be either guaiac-based or immunochemical.[20] If unusual FOBT results are found, members are normally alluded for a subsequent colonoscopy assessment. Whenever done once every 1-2 years, FOBT screening diminishes colorectal malignant growth passings by 16% and among those partaking in screening, colorectal disease passings can be decreased up to 23%, despite the fact that it has not been demonstrated to lessen all-cause mortality.[121] Immunochemical tests are precise and don't need dietary or prescription changes before testing. Nonetheless, research in the UK has found that for these immunochemical tests, the limit for additional examination is set at a point that might miss the greater part of entrail malignant growth cases. The exploration proposes that the NHS Britain's Gut Malignant growth Screening System could utilize the test's capacity to give the specific grouping of blood in defecation (as opposed to just whether it is above or under an end level).

Different choices incorporate virtual colonoscopy and stool DNA screening testing (FIT-DNA). Virtual colonoscopy by means of a CT examine shows up comparable to standard colonoscopy for distinguishing diseases and huge adenomas yet is costly, related with radiation openness, and can't eliminate any identified unusual developments as standard colonoscopy can.[20] Stool DNA screening test searches for biomarkers related with colorectal malignant growth and precancerous injuries, including modified DNA and blood hemoglobin. A positive outcome ought to be trailed by colonoscopy. FIT-DNA has more bogus up-sides than FIT and consequently brings about more unfriendly effects.[10] Further review is expected starting around 2016 to decide if a three-year screening span is right.

Suggestions

In the US, screening is commonly suggested between ages 50 and 75 years.[10][125] The American Disease Society suggests beginning at the period of 45.[126] For those somewhere in the range of 76 and 85 years of age, the choice to screen ought to be individualized.[10] For those at high gamble, screenings as a rule start at around 40.[20][127]

A few screening techniques are suggested including stool-based tests like clockwork, sigmoidoscopy like clockwork with waste immunochemical testing at regular intervals, and colonoscopy each 10 years.[125] It is hazy which of these two strategies is better.[128] Colonoscopy might track down additional malignant growths in the initial segment of the colon, yet is related with more noteworthy expense and more complications.[128] For individuals with normal gamble who have had an excellent colonoscopy with typical outcomes, the American Gastroenterological Affiliation suggests no sort of separating the 10 years following the colonoscopy.[129][130] For individuals more than 75 or those with a future of under 10 years, screening isn't recommended.[131] It requires around 10 years in the wake of evaluating for one out of a 1000 group to benefit.[132] The USPSTF list seven expected methodologies for screening, with the main thing being that no less than one of these procedures is properly used.[10]

In Canada, among those 50 to 75 years of age at typical gamble, waste immunochemical testing or FOBT is suggested like clockwork or sigmoidoscopy each 10 years.[133] Colonoscopy is less preferred.[133]

A few nations have public colorectal evaluating programs which offer FOBT evaluating for all grown-ups inside a specific age bunch, ordinarily beginning between ages 50 and 60. Instances of nations with coordinated screening incorporate the Unified Kingdom,[134] Australia,[135] the Netherlands,[136] Hong Kong, and Taiwan.

The UK Entrail Disease Screening Project means to find advance notice signs in individuals matured 60 to 74, by suggesting a waste immunochemical test (FIT) like clockwork. FIT estimates blood in defecation, and individuals with levels over a specific edge might have entrail tissue analyzed for indications of malignant growth. Developments having dangerous potential are removed.

Treatment

The therapy of colorectal malignant growth can be focused on fix or concealment. The choice on which plan to take on relies upon different variables, including the individual's wellbeing and inclinations, as well as the phase of the tumor.[139] Evaluation in multidisciplinary groups is a basic piece of deciding if the patient is reasonable for medical procedure or not.[140] When colorectal disease is gotten early, medical procedure can be healing. In any case, when it is distinguished at later stages (for which metastases are available), this is more uncertain and treatment is frequently aimed at concealment, to alleviate side effects brought about by the growth and keep the individual as agreeable as possible.

Medical procedure

At a beginning phase, colorectal malignant growth might be eliminated during a colonoscopy utilizing one of a few methods, including endoscopic mucosal resection or endoscopic submucosal dissection.[5] Endoscopic resection is conceivable on the off chance that there is low chance of lymph hub metastasis and the size and area of the growth make en coalition resection possible.[141] For individuals with restricted disease, the favored treatment is finished careful evacuation with satisfactory edges, with the endeavor of accomplishing a fix. The technique of decision is an incomplete colectomy (or proctocolectomy for rectal injuries) where the impacted piece of the colon or rectum is eliminated alongside parts of its mesocolon and blood supply to work with evacuation of depleting lymph hubs. This should be possible either by an open laparotomy or laparoscopically, contingent upon factors connected with the unique individual and injury factors.[20]

The colon may then be reconnected or an individual might have a colostomy.[5]

On the off chance that there are a couple of metastases in the liver or lungs, these may likewise be eliminated. Chemotherapy might be utilized before a medical procedure to shrivel the malignant growth prior to endeavoring to eliminate it. The two most normal locales of repeat of colorectal malignant growth are the liver and lungs. For peritoneal carcinomatosis cytoreductive medical procedure, some of the time in blend with HIPEC can be utilized trying to eliminate the cancer.

Chemotherapy

In both malignant growth of the colon and rectum, chemotherapy might be utilized notwithstanding a medical procedure in specific cases. The choice to add chemotherapy in administration of colon and rectal malignant growth relies upon the phase of the disease.

In Stage I colon disease, no chemotherapy is offered, and medical procedure is the authoritative therapy. The job of chemotherapy in Stage II colon disease is disputable, and is generally not offered except if risk factors like T4 cancer, undifferentiated growth, vascular and perineural attack or lacking lymph hub examining is identified.[144] It is additionally realized that individuals who convey anomalies of the confuse fix qualities don't profit from chemotherapy. For Stage III and Stage IV colon malignant growth, chemotherapy is an indispensable piece of treatment.

Assuming disease has spread to the lymph hubs or far off organs, which is the situation with Stage III and Stage IV colon malignant growth separately, adding chemotherapy specialists fluorouracil, capecitabine or oxaliplatin increments future. In the event that the lymph hubs don't contain disease, the advantages of chemotherapy are disputable. In the event that the disease is broadly metastatic or unrespectable, treatment is palliative. Normally here, various different chemotherapy prescriptions might be used.[20] Chemotherapy drugs for this condition might incorporate capecitabine, fluorouracil, irinotecan, oxaliplatin and UFT.[145] The medications capecitabine and fluorouracil are tradable, with capecitabine being an oral drug and fluorouracil being an intravenous medication. A few explicit regimens utilized for CRC are CAPOX, FOLFOX, FOLFOXIRI, and FOLFIRI.[146] Antiangiogenic medications, for example, bevacizumab are many times included first line therapy.[citation needed] One more class of medications utilized in the subsequent line setting are epidermal development factor receptor inhibitors, of which the three FDA supported ones are aflibercept, cetuximab and panitumumab.[147][148]

The essential distinction in the way to deal with low stage rectal malignant growth is the fuse of radiation treatment. Frequently, it is utilized related to chemotherapy in a neoadjuvant design to empower careful resection, with the goal that at last a colostomy isn't needed. Be that as it may, it may not be imaginable in low lying cancers, in which case, a long-lasting colostomy might be required. Stage IV rectal disease is dealt with like Stage IV colon malignant growth.

Stage IV colorectal malignant growth due to peritoneal carcinomatosis can be dealt with utilizing HIPEC joined with cytoreductive medical procedure.

Radiation treatment

While a mix of radiation and chemotherapy might be helpful for rectal cancer,[20] for certain individuals requiring therapy, chemoradiotherapy can increment intense therapy related harmfulness, and has not been displayed to further develop endurance rates contrasted with radiotherapy alone, in spite of the fact that it is related with less nearby recurrence.[142] The utilization of radiotherapy in colon malignant growth isn't normal because of the responsiveness of the guts to radiation.[153] Similarly as with chemotherapy, radiotherapy can be utilized as a neoadjuvant for clinical stages T3 and T4 for rectal cancer.[154] This outcomes in scaling back or down staging of the growth, setting it up for careful resection, and furthermore diminishes neighbourhood repeat rates.[154] For privately progressed rectal disease, neoadjuvant chemo radiotherapy has turned into the standard treatment.[155] Moreover, when medical procedure is preposterous radiation treatment has been proposed to be a viable therapy against CRC pneumonic metastases, which are created by 10-15% of individuals with CRC.

Immunotherapy

Immunotherapy with invulnerable designated spot inhibitors has been viewed as valuable for a sort of colorectal disease with confuse fix inadequacy and microsatellite instability.[157][158][159] Pembrolizumab is supported for cutting edge CRC cancers that are MMR insufficient and have fizzled common treatments.[160] The vast majority who do improve, in any case, actually deteriorate after months or years.[158]

Then again, in a planned stage 2 review distributed in June 2022 in The New Britain Diary of Medication, 12 patients with Lacking Jumble Fix (dMMR) stage II or III rectal adenocarcinoma were managed single-specialist dostarlimab, an enemy of PD-1 monoclonal immunizer, like clockwork for quite a long time. After a middle development of a year (range, 6 to 25 months), each of the 12 patients had a total clinical reaction without any proof of growth on X-ray, 18F-fluorodeoxyglucose-positron-outflow tomography, endoscopic assessment, computerized rectal assessment, or biopsy. Additionally, no tolerant in the preliminary required chemoradiotherapy or medical procedure, and no understanding revealed antagonistic occasions of grade 3 or higher. Notwithstanding, albeit the consequences of this study are promising, the review is little and has vulnerabilities about long haul outcomes.[161]

Palliative consideration

Palliative consideration is suggested for any individual who has progressed colon disease or who has huge symptoms.[162][163]

Association of palliative consideration might be useful to work on the personal satisfaction for both the individual and their family, by further developing side effects, tension and forestalling admissions to the hospital.

In individuals with hopeless colorectal disease, palliative consideration can comprise of methodology that alleviate side effects or complexities from the malignant growth yet don't endeavor to fix the basic disease, consequently working on personal satisfaction. Careful choices might incorporate non-remedial careful expulsion of a portion of the malignant growth tissue, bypassing part of the digestion tracts, or stent situation. These techniques can be considered to further develop side effects and lessen intricacies like draining from the growth, stomach torment and digestive obstruction.[165] Non-employable strategies for suggestive therapy incorporate radiation treatment to diminish growth size as well as agony medications.[166]

Follow-up

The U.S. Public Far reaching Disease Organization and American Culture of Clinical Oncology give rules to the development of colon cancer.[167][168] A clinical history and actual assessment are prescribed each 3 to a half year for a long time, then at regular intervals for quite a long time. Carcinoembryonic antigen blood level estimations follow a similar timing, however are just exhorted for individuals with T2 or more noteworthy sores who are possibility for mediation. A CT-output of the chest, mid-region and pelvis can be thought about every year for the initial 3 years for individuals who are at high gamble of repeat (for instance, the people who had inadequately separated growths or venous or lymphatic intrusion) and are possibility for corrective medical procedure (with the mean to fix). A colonoscopy should be possible following 1 year, with the exception of in the event that it wasn't possible during the underlying organizing due to a deterring mass, in which case it ought to be performed following 3 to a half year. If a villous polyp, a polyp >1 centimeter or high-grade dysplasia is found, it very well may be rehashed following 3 years, then at regular intervals. For different anomalies, the colonoscopy can be rehashed after 1 year.

Routine PET or ultrasound filtering, chest X-beams, complete blood count or liver capability tests are not recommended.

For individuals who have gone through healing a medical procedure or adjuvant treatment (or both) to treat non-metastatic colorectal malignant growth, extraordinary observation and close subsequent have not been displayed to give extra endurance benefits.

Work out

Exercise might be suggested in the future as auxiliary treatment to malignant growth survivors. In epidemiological examinations, exercise might diminish colorectal malignant growth explicit mortality and all-cause mortality. Results for the particular measures of activity expected to notice an advantage were clashing. These distinctions might reflect contrasts in cancer science and the outflow of biomarkers. Individuals with growths that needed CTNNB1 articulation (β-catenin), associated with Wnt flagging pathway, required in excess of 18 metabolic same (MET) hours of the week, a proportion of activity, to notice a decrease in colorectal disease mortality. The component of how exercise benefits endurance might be associated with resistant observation and irritation pathways. In clinical examinations, a favorable to fiery reaction was found in individuals with stage II-III colorectal malignant growth who went through about fourteen days of moderate activity subsequent to finishing their essential treatment. Oxidative equilibrium might be one more conceivable instrument for benefits noticed.

A critical decline in 8-oxo-dG was found in the pee of individuals who went through about fourteen days of moderate activity after essential treatment. Other potential components might include metabolic chemical and sex-steroid chemicals, albeit these pathways might be engaged with different sorts of cancers.

Another potential biomarker might be p27. Survivors with growths that communicated p27 and performed more prominent and equivalent to 18 MET hours of the week were found to have decreased colorectal disease mortality endurance contrasted with those with under 18 MET hours out of every week. Survivors without p27 articulation who practiced were displayed to have more awful results. The constitutive actuation of PI3K/AKT/mTOR pathway might make sense of the deficiency of p27 and abundance energy equilibrium might up-control p27 to prevent disease cells from dividing.

Active work gives advantages to individuals non-progressed colorectal malignant growth. Upgrades in oxygen consuming wellness, malignant growth related weakness and wellbeing related personal satisfaction have been accounted for in the short term.[172] Nonetheless, these enhancements were not seen at the degree of illness related emotional well-being, like tension and depression.

Guess

Less than 600 qualities are connected to results in colorectal cancer.[51] These incorporate the two negative qualities, where high articulation is connected with unfortunate result, for instance the intensity shock 70 kDa protein 1 (HSPA1A), and great qualities where high articulation is related with better endurance, for instance the putative RNA-restricting protein 3

(RBM3).[51] The guess is likewise corresponded with an unfortunate devotion of the pre-mRNA grafting contraption, and subsequently countless veering off elective splicing.[173]

Repeat rates

Primary article: Malignant growth repeat § Rectal disease

The typical five-year repeat rate in individuals where medical procedure is fruitful is 5% for stage I malignant growths, 12% in stage II and 33% in stage III. Be that as it may, contingent upon the quantity of chance variables it goes from 9-22% in stage II and 17-44% in stage III.

Endurance rates

In Europe the five-year endurance rate for colorectal malignant growth is under 60%. In the created world about 33% of individuals who get the illness bite the dust from it.

Endurance is straightforwardly connected with discovery and the kind of disease included, however generally is poor for indicative malignant growths, as they are normally much progressed. Endurance rates for beginning phase recognition are multiple times that of late stage diseases. Individuals with a growth that has not penetrated the muscularis mucosa (TNM stage Tis, N0, M0) have a five-year endurance pace of 100 percent, while those with obtrusive disease of T1 (inside the submucosal layer) or T2 (inside the strong layer) have a typical five-year endurance pace of roughly

90%. Those with a more intrusive cancer yet without hub inclusion (T3-4, N0, M0) have a typical five-year endurance pace of roughly 70%. Individuals with positive provincial lymph hubs (any T, N1-3, M0) have a typical five-year endurance pace of roughly 40%, while those with far off metastases (any T, any N, M1) have an unfortunate visualization and the long term endurance goes from <5 percent to 31 percent. The forecast relies upon a large number of variables which incorporate the actual wellness level of the individual, degree of metastases, and cancer grade.

While the effect of colorectal malignant growth on the individuals who endure differs enormously there will frequently be a need to adjust to both physical and mental results of the disease and its treatment.[180] For instance, it is normal for individuals to encounter incontinence,[181] sexual dysfunction,[182] issues with stoma care[183] and apprehension about disease recurrence[184] after essential treatment has closed.

A subjective methodical survey distributed in 2021 featured that there are three primary variables impacting transformation to living with and past colorectal disease: support components, seriousness of late impacts of treatment and psychosocial change. In this manner, fundamental individuals are offered suitable help to assist them with better adjusting to life following treatment.[185]

The study of disease transmission

Starting around 2012, it is the second most normal reason for disease in ladies (9.2% of analyses) and the third most normal in men (10.0%)[14]: 16 with it being the fourth most normal reason for malignant growth demise after lung, stomach, and liver cancer.[187] It is more normal in created than creating countries.[188] Worldwide occurrence shifts 10-overlap, with most noteworthy rates in Australia, New Zealand, Europe and the US and least rates in Africa and South-Focal Asia.

US

In 2022, the frequency of colorectal malignant growth in the US was expected to be around 151,000 grown-ups, including more than 106,000 new instances of colon disease (nearly 54,000 men and 52,000 ladies) and around 45,000 new instances of rectal cancer.[190] Since the 1980s, the occurrence of colorectal disease diminished, coming around 2% every year from 2014 to 2018 in grown-ups matured 50 and more seasoned, due principally to improved screening.[190] Notwithstanding, rate of colorectal malignant growth has expanded in people matured 25 to 50. In mid 2023, the American Malignant growth Society (ACS) announced that 20% of determinations (of colon malignant growth) in 2019 were in patients under age 55, which is about twofold the rate in 1995, and paces of cutting edge illness expanded by around 3% yearly in individuals more youthful than 50. That's what it anticipated, in 2023, an expected 19,550 judgments and 3,750 passings would be in individuals more youthful than 50.[191] Colorectal disease additionally excessively influences the African American population, where the rates are the most noteworthy of any racial/ethnic gathering in the US. African Americans are around 20% bound to get colorectal disease and around 40% bound to kick the bucket from it than most different gatherings. Dark Americans frequently experience more prominent obstructions to malignant growth avoidance, identification, therapy, and endurance, including foundational racial abberations that are perplexing and go past the conspicuous association with disease.

Papua New Guinea

In the emerging nations like Papua New Guinea and other Pacific Island States including the Solomon Islands, colorectal malignant growth is an exceptionally uncommon disease among individuals, which is least normal contrasted with lung, stomach, liver or bosom disease. It is assessed that no less than 8 out of 100,000 individuals are probably going to created colorectal disease each year, which is not normal for lung or bosom malignant growth, where for the last option alone is 24 out of 100,000 ladies.

Techniques: Patients more than 65-year-old determined to have colorectal malignant growth somewhere in the range of 2000 and 2014 were separated from Observation, The study of disease transmission, and Final products (Soothsayer) connected data set.

Results: A sum of 136,872 patients with colorectal disease met the incorporation models. The middle subsequent time was around 3 years. 45 point seven percent of them were alive toward the finish of follow-up, colorectal malignant growth actually represented the most instances of passings. Nonetheless, patients with growth of Grade I or TNM stage I-II were bound to kick the bucket from different causes. The completely changed relative perils proportion (HR) shows age, orientation, growth site, chemotherapy, cancer qualities of grade and TNM stage impacted the two sorts of mortality. Race just impacted mortality of different causes. Cardiovascular sickness (CVD) was a recognizable reason for death among patients with stage I colorectal malignant growth. With longer development, passings because of colorectal malignant growth diminished while passings of CVD, aspiratory sicknesses and other reason for death expanded.

Ends: Colorectal disease actually represents most passings in old patients. Nonetheless, comorbidities including CVD/COPD were related with the passings of colorectal disease patients more than 65. As endurance time builds, comorbidities ought to be considered for malignant growth treatment. The board of CVD/COPD among older patients can assist with working on in general endurance (operating system) in colorectal malignant growth.

Leading epidemiologic examination on malignant growth survivorship depends on all-cause mortality, and that implies the most ordinarily involved result in clinical examinations for colorectal disease is the amount of colorectal disease explicit mortality and mortality of different causes. Evaluation of results for both colorectal disease explicit mortality and mortality of different causes can help specialists in finding prognostic pointers and selecting the main clinical consideration to work on patients' endurance. This study displayed elements of colorectal disease explicit mortality and other mortality and investigated the main source of death among colorectal malignant growth patients from the Observation, The study of disease transmission, and Outcome (Soothsayer) information base.

Methods other Area

Patient choice

Information of the ongoing concentrate on the patients with colorectal disease somewhere in the range of 2000 and 2014 was recovered from the Soothsayer data set. Supported by the Public Disease Foundation, the Soothsayer data set covers 26% populace from 18 disease libraries of USA with both occurrence and endurance data of malignancies.

Data of both treatment subtleties and clinicopathological factors were separated. Patients north of 65 years of age who met the accompanying standards were incorporated: (I) patients were obsessively determined to have colorectal malignant growth; (II) colorectal disease was the main essential carcinoma. Patients with fragmented TNM arranging or endurance information were prohibited.

Measurable dissect

The review partners were separated into three subgroups: (I) patients who were alive during our review period; (II) patients who kicked the bucket because of colorectal disease explicit causes toward the finish of the review time frame; (III) patients who passed on from different causes. For additional examination of other-reasons for death, we ordered other-cause mortality into three gatherings: the cardiovascular illness (CVD), pneumonic infections including constant obstructive aspiratory sickness (COPD) and others.

For portraying the clinicopathological qualities of associates, quantitative qualities and medians with interquartile ranges (IQRs) were used. Multivariate Cox relative danger relapse models were built after univariate Cox corresponding peril relapse models to decide the relationship between trademark variables and endurance status. Endurance bends of 4 gatherings with various age ranges were drawn utilizing the Kaplan-Meier technique. Contrasts in endurance were analyzed by the Log-rank test. Growth stage was coded in light of the UICC/AJCC TNM organizing framework (eighth version). The endpoints in light old enough at analysis sprang from past review.

R programming for Windows (adaptation R-3.4.3, the R Starting point for factual processing) was performed for all measurable examinations. All factual examinations were two sided. Furthermore, a P<0.05 was evaluated as an edge of factual importance.

Results Other Area

A sum of 136,872 patients who met the consideration measures were remembered for our companions. Among these patients, 74,307 people (54.3%) passed on during the review time frame: 45,131 (33.0%) of the review companions kicked the bucket because of colorectal disease, while the other 29,176 (21.3%) passed on because of different causes. Among them, 14,489 patients passed on from CVD and 2,413 passed on from COPD or other aspiratory sicknesses. The middle subsequent time was 37 months

(IQR: 13-74), and the middle age at death was 79 years of age (IQR: 72-84). By and large, colorectal malignant growth actually represented the most instances of passings while patients with cancer of Grade I or TNM stage I-II were bound to bite the dust from non-tumorous causes (Table 1).

Clinicopathological attributes in three subgroups of mortality status in colorectal disease patients north of 65-year-old in Soothsayer data set

Both the age-changed relative dangers proportion (HR) of death actuated by colorectal malignant growth and different causes were more noteworthy among patients with old age, male patients, treatment with chemoradiotherapy and higher TNM stage. After change for age, TNM stage, histopathologic grade, growth site and remedial plans, HR of colorectal disease explicit mortality was not the same as mortality of other-causes. Age, orientation, cancer site, chemotherapy, growth qualities of grade and TNM stage impacted the two sorts of mortality, while race just impacted mortality of other-causes.

Age-changed and multivariate examination of colorectal disease mortality and other-cause mortality in patients north of 65-year-old in Soothsayer data set

The extent of various reasons for death was different by age and cancer stages. Patients experienced growth with higher stages were significantly more prone to kick the bucket because of colorectal disease rather than different causes. Then again, different reasons for death happened more probable among patients with stage I-II malignant growths. In subgroups of various age ranges, CVD represented the most noteworthy extent of passings among patients determined to have stage I colorectal malignant growth. CVD was additionally the subsequent driving reason for passings for patients with stage II-IV colorectal disease. Inside all stages, there was expanding extent of other-causes passings as patients matured.

Extent of various driving reasons for death in colorectal malignant growth patients more than 65 of subgroups separated by age at conclusion and by phase of sickness.

The extent of combined reasons for death was likewise subject to the length of follow-up time. With longer development, the extent of passings because of colorectal malignant growth diminished while passings of CVD, aspiratory sicknesses and different reasons for death expanded persistently. Different reasons for death in this class included passings brought about by Alzheimer's sickness (n=1,498, 1.09%) and diabetes (n=1,081, 0.79%).

Changing appropriation of aggregate reasons for death by time since colorectal malignant growth analysis.

Discussion Other Segment

In our clinical practice, an ever increasing number of old patients with colorectal malignant growth get a medical procedure or potentially chemoradiotherapy. Meanwhile, they are bound to have comorbidities, like CVD, pneumonic infection (like COPD and flu), making treatment more dangerous (9). As per logical measurements, age is an autonomous prognostic component for both in-medical clinic dreariness and mortality after colorectal medical procedure (10,11). Subsequently, we generally hold a negative demeanor towards the therapy of colorectal malignant growth in old patients (12). In clinical practice, we lean toward surrender a medical procedure or decline chemotherapy portion, since we have a conventional thought that older patients may not pass on from colorectal disease but rather from comorbidities. Be that as it may, in our partner, we tracked down just patients with early grade growth, and beginning phase were bound to bite the dust because of different causes, while colorectal disease actually represented most passings in old patients. Subsequently, we advocate dynamic enemy of growth treatment for older patients with colorectal disease.

Patients with early grade cancer and beginning phase were bound to pass on because of different causes. For these patients, notwithstanding against growth treatment, we ought to put more consideration on infections of different causes, like CVD, COPD and other lung illnesses. In our review, CVD was shown as the subsequent driving reason for death in our partners (n=14,489, 10.59%), second just to colorectal malignant growth (n=45,131, 32.97%). Also, particularly in patients with stage I colorectal disease, CVD was the essential driver of death. This is on the grounds that patients north of 65 have a higher rate of comorbidities and patients with comorbidities are bound to kick the bucket because of different causes. At the point when patients endure longer, CVD might turn into the main source of death.

In both HR of colorectal disease mortality and other-cause mortality, men are altogether more in danger than ladies. This can be made sense of by a few reasons. To begin with, estrogen defensively affects colorectal disease in ladies, and ladies have a 7-8 years slack in creating colorectal malignant growth (13). Second, with regards to way of life and wellbeing, ladies are without a doubt better than men overall. Smoking and drinking are still vices that numerous male patients with colorectal disease can't dispose of. Third, in both east and west, men are still commonly given more liability than ladies. Along with the general public's 'meaning' of male jobs, men actually will quite often be more forceful and persevere through issues regardless of whether they can't hang on. These are not just awful for their physical and emotional well-being, yet additionally terrible for early recognition and analysis.

Ethnic contrasts additionally frequently influence treatment choice. For the most part, white patients have relative low perils of colorectal malignant growth passings than dark patients. Be that as it may, for different reasons for passings, there was no factual distinction between these two races. Since colorectal malignant growth occurrence and mortality are declining throughout the last many years attributable to the reception of successful screening programs (14), we point out for more colorectal disease separating individuals of color to kill the distinction in mortality.

As far as growth site, we can see that the endurance of left colon disease is somewhat more awful than that of right colon malignant growth regarding both colorectal malignant growth passing and other-causes demise. This is in opposition to other writing, which advocates that because of contrasts in undeveloped organism beginning, physical design and physiological capability, right colon malignant growth might have more regrettable natural way of behaving (15). In any case, different examinations likewise have shown no massive contrast in generally speaking endurance (operating system) and illness free endurance (DFS) after medical procedure for left and right colon malignant growth, and the operating system and DFS for early right colon disease are higher than those for left colon malignant growth (15). Since stage IV patients represented just a little part of our review companion, it is sensible to accept that the endurance of patients with right colon disease might be preferable over those with left colon malignant growth.

In HR of colorectal disease mortality, we found that in age-changed model, chemoradiotherapy is a gamble factor for colorectal malignant growth passing. Notwithstanding, after completely changed by age, growth stage, grade, site and therapies, chemoradiotherapy turns into a defensive variable for colorectal disease passing. This can be made sense of by the way that for all patients, chemoradiotherapy frequently includes patients with late stage and inadequately separated growths, so chemoradiotherapy is a gamble factor; yet after changed by all elements, for patients with similar stage and qualities, chemoradiotherapy offers a preferred endurance over denying it.

Growth grade is a gamble factor for colorectal disease demise, yet not impact the other reason for death. Be that as it may, TNM organizing is a gamble factor for both colorectal disease passing and other reason for death.

This is on the grounds that the seriousness of colorectal malignant growth will likewise influence non-neoplastic sicknesses, particularly for patients with metastasis who need extraordinary chemoradiotherapy, and so on. The results of chemoradiotherapy will likewise build the predominance of comorbidities.

Obviously, our review is pretty much flawed, which is restricted by the legitimacy of death coding. The legitimacy of reason for death affirmation isn't altogether exact, which has been found to fluctuate in various malignant growth site, season of conclusion and ages at death (16). Likewise, the Framingham Heart Study (17) have shown that coronary illness might be over-assessed in genuine conclusion for the reason for death for the most part. Thus, the paces of CVD might be misjudged in this study populace determined to have colorectal malignant growth. Moreover, there are various definitely missing records for race, grade and medical procedure status. This data might impact the finish of our review. All in all, colorectal malignant growth actually represents most passings in old patients. Be that as it may, older patients are related with expanding hazard of mortality from other comorbidities, particularly CVD and pneumonic illnesses. Patients with Grade I growth and TNM stage I-II were bound to kick the bucket because of different causes as opposed to colorectal disease. As endurance time increments, passings because of colorectal malignant growth decline while passings of CVD, pneumonic sicknesses increment. Thus, we ought to in any case send off dynamic enemy of growth treatment for old patients with colorectal disease, yet for beginning phase cancers and as patients live longer, therapy of other existing comorbidities ought to likewise be considered into the timetable of patients' administration. Particularly among colorectal malignant growth survivors north of 65, legitimate administration of CVD/COPD might work on patients' operating system.

Different pathways interceding the inception, movement, and relocation of CRC, like Wnt/β-catenin, Indent, Hedgehog, and TGF-β (changing development factor-β)/SMAD, as well as those equipped for initiating flagging fountains, for example, phosphatidylinositol 3-kinase (PI3K)/AKT or RAS/quickly sped up fibrosarcoma (RAF), contain ideal destinations for designated treatment (Fig. 2).27,28 Given the complex downstream flagging and troubles in totally hindering explicit natural collaborations, not all current CRC-related pathways can be effectively obstructed, and current information cover a couple of pathways in which tentatively distinguished designated specialists can be ended up being proficient in clinical examinations, and an enormous gathering of designated drugs stay in preclinical status or in stage I preliminaries.

CHAPTER 4

FOCUSING ON ANGIOGENESIS

Bevacizumab: the achievement

The milestone preliminaries in light of antiangiogenic treatment for CRC were started in 2004, containing the stage II and III AVF2107 preliminaries, which affirmed the predominance of chemotherapy (IRI, 5-FU, and leucovorin) in addition to bevacizumab over chemotherapy in addition to placebo.182 Bevacizumab is a refined IgG monoclonal immune response designated to VEGF-A that, as per the AVF2107 preliminary, works on both PFS and operating system in metastatic CRC (RR: 44% versus 34.8%; operating system: 20.3 versus 15.6 months; HR: 0.66, p < 0.001; PFS: 10.6 versus 6.2 months; HR: 0.54; p < 0.001). In this way, the FDA-endorsed bevacizumab as the main VEGF-designated specialist for metastatic CRC, despite the fact that few preliminaries researching bevacizumab in addition to immunotherapy or FOLFOX/FOXFIRI showed just a fractional huge improvement in one or the other operating system or PFS.182,183,184,185,186,187 Utilizing bevacizumab may prompt 10% more grade 3-5 unfriendly occasions, like hypertension or leukopenia,188 while it remained somewhat protected and powerful while treating old patients with CRC (mature more than 70 years of age) in the stage III AVEX trial.185 Further examination found that the two patients with KRAS changes and those with a wild-type genotype might profit from bevacizumab.189,190,191 Both left-and right-sided colon cancers answer well to bevacizumab.191 Two free preliminaries expressed no distinction as far as viability against metastatic CRC among FOLFOX and FOLFIRI joined with bevacizumab.192,193 Yet curiously, a bevacizumab-containing routine appeared to have improved adequacy with the trio FOLFOXIRI routine than FOLFIRI alone (PFS: 12.3 versus 9.7 months; HR: 0.77; p =

0.006; operating system: 29.8 versus 25.8 months; HR: 0.80; p = 0.03), albeit the last doublet routine had less unfavourable responses as per the Clan trial.187

Notwithstanding first-line use of bevacizumab, different preliminaries have approved its adequacy in the second-line setting. Longer PFS (7.3 versus 4.7 months, HR = 0.61, p < 0.001) and operating system (12.9 versus 10.8 months, HR = 0.75, p = 0.0011), as well as a superior reaction rate (22.7% versus 8.6%, p = 0.0001), were found in the E3200 preliminary with a mix of FOLFOX and bevacizumab than with FOLFOX alone for patients with CRC who advanced after FOLFOX therapy.194 Comparative mathematical contrasts were likewise noted in the correlation with bevacizumab alone. All things being equal, continuation on bevacizumab for the individuals who advanced after first-line chemotherapy was as yet supportive for PFS (5.7 versus 4.1 months, HR = 0.68, p < 0.001) and operating system (11.2 versus 9.9 months, HR = 0.81, p = 0.0062) improvement contrasted and standard chemotherapy alone in the stage III ML18147 trial.195

As far as upkeep, or at least, bevacizumab after first-line chemotherapy in stable CRC, a progression of preliminaries showed that enemy of VEGF specialists may be very appealing. The imminent and observational BRiTE concentrate on showed that bevacizumab continuation decisively worked on the operating system of patients with CRC (31.8 versus 19.9 months, HR = 0.48, p < 0.001) in correlation with no maintenance.196 Continuation of CAP and bevacizumab altogether delayed the movement time in patients after first-line XELOX in addition to bevacizumab contrasted and perception

(11.7 versus 8.5 months, HR = 0.67, p < 0.0001)186 paying little mind to RAS/BRAF change status and confuse fix (MMR) status.197

Patterns of longer operating system (23.2 versus 20.0 months, HR = 1.05, p = 0.65 in the Large scale preliminary and 25.4 versus 23.8 months, HR = 0.83, p = 0.2 in the SAKK (Swiss Gathering for Clinical Disease Exploration) preliminary) have been noticed for upkeep bevacizumab in addition to XELOX over bevacizumab alone in the Large scale trial198 and for keeping up with single-specialist bevacizumab treatment contrasted and no treatment in the SAKK trial.199 No mediocrity has been found for support of bevacizumab alone over bevacizumab in addition to 5-FU or continuation of bevacizumab in addition to Cover over bevacizumab in addition to XELOX.200,201

Arising against VEGFR specialists

As of recently, just bevacizumab has been FDA endorsed as a first-and second-line VEGF-designated specialist for CRC, albeit different novel specialists are arising, and some of them have been supported for second-line treatment of CRC.

Aflibercept is a VEGFR-1 and VEGFR-2 extracellular space recombinant combination protein that goes about as a ligand trap focusing on VEGF-A, VEGF-B, and PIGF. Aflibercept has a more grounded fondness for VEGF-A than bevacizumab.202 The single-specialist advantage of aflibercept is by all accounts limited,202 while chemo-blends showed extraordinary potential as per the stage III Courage preliminary, wherein the expansion of aflibercept after Bull or bevacizumab in metastatic CRC patients getting FOXFIRI acquired a superior reaction (19.8% versus 11.1%) as well as a more extended PFS (6.9 versus 4.7 months, HR = 0.76; p < 0.001) and operating system (13.5 versus 12.1 months, HR = 0.82; p = 0.0032) than FOXFIRI in addition to placebo.203 Nonetheless, as far as the first-line setting, as in the stage II Certify preliminary, the blend of aflibercept with FOLFOX didn't bring about recognizable advantages in PFS or reaction rate, however brought about expanded unfavourable occasion rates. Subsequently, aflibercept ought to stay a second-line suggested CRC agent.204

Ramucirumab, a completely refined monoclonal VEGFR-2-designated IgG immunizer, is another FDA-endorsed drug for second-line treatment of metastatic CRC in view of the stage III RAISE preliminary. In this second-line-setting preliminary, a blend of ramucirumab and FOLFIRI fundamentally delayed PFS (5.7 versus 4.5 months; HR = 0.79, p < .0005) and operating system (13.3 versus 11.7 months, HR = 0.84, p = 0.022) contrasted with FOLFIRI-placebo.205 Comparative with the discoveries with aflibercept, a stage II preliminary showed that the FOLFOX routine may not profit from expansion to ramucirumab concerning PFS.206

TKIs have turned into an engaging decision for patients with against EGFR-safe NSCLC, while in patients with CRC, not very many medications have shown to be compelling. Regorafenib, a TKI with different targets, like VEGFR, PDGFR (platelet-determined development factor receptor), FGFR (fibroblast development factor receptor), and BRAF, was endorsed by the

FDA to treat metastatic CRC. A first-line study concerning regorafenib in addition to FOLFOX in CRC found no improvement in the reaction rate contrasted and FOLFOX in addition to placebo.207 In any case, for headstrong metastatic CRC treatment, in the stage III Right trial,208 better middle operating system (6.4 versus 5.0 months, HR = 0.77, p = 0.0052) and PFS (1.9 versus 1.7 months, HR = 0.49, p < 0.0001) were accomplished utilizing regorafenib than utilizing fake treatment, which has additionally been approved in an Asian populace in the Agree preliminary (PFS: 3.2 versus 1.7 months, HR = 0.31, p < 0.0001; operating system: 8.8 versus 6.3 months, HR = 0.55, p = 0.0002).209

Different specialists are being grown rapidly. The stage III FRESCO preliminary upheld fruquintinib, a TKI with the capacity to hinder VEGFR-1, VEGFR-2, and VEGFR-3, as a suggested decision for chemotherapy against obstinate metastatic CRC. In this Chinese-based study, operating system (9.3 versus 6.6 months, HR = 0.65, p < 0.001) and PFS (3.7 versus 1.8 months, HR = 0.26, p < 0.001) were essentially delayed with fruquintinib contrasted with placebo,210 which drove with endorsement of by the China Food and Medication Organization (CFDA) otherwise called NMPA (Public Clinical Items Organization). Famitinib is another TKI focusing on the c-Unit receptor, VEGFR-2, and VEGFR-3, PDGFR, and RET that is being examined in a continuous stage II review, which has so far shown a superior PFS (2.8 versus 1.5 months, HR = 0.58, p = 0.0034) and infectious prevention rate (57.58% versus 30.91%, p = 0.0023) for Famitinib, with results concerning operating system standing by to be reported.211

New TKIs communicating noteworthy antitumor impacts in preclinical examinations have delivered uninspiring operating system and RR values in late reports; in any case, PFS might be drawn out by medications, for example, the VEGFR-2-and FGFR-focused on brivanib212 and cediranib, a TKI designated to each of the three VEGFRs and PDGFR that neglected to introduce viability towards CRC control in the stage II and III Skyline study,213,214 as did nintedanib, a TKI with the capacity to impede all VEGFRs, FGFR1-3, PDGFR-α, and PDGFR-β, as per the stage III LUME-Colon 1 trial.215 Other on-market TKIs, for example, the gastrointestinal stromal cancer (Significance)- focused on imatinib and sunitinib and the squamous cell carcinoma-targeted erlotinib and gefitinib, have no indication or supporting data for treating CRC.

Focusing on the HGF/c-MET pathway

Gathering information on the cozy connection among disease and the HGF-MET pathway distinguishes it as a profoundly encouraging site for designated treatment. Different approaches to obstructing HGF-MET by means of recently evolved monoclonal antibodies or little particles with various pharmacological components have arisen. For HGF, drugs are focused on either impeding HGF actuation and creation or slowing down the limiting of HGF to MET receptors. In the last option case, specialists either seriously tie to MET receptors (MET adversaries) or restrain intracellular tyrosine kinase movement (MET TKIs). Until this point, no serious unfriendly occasions have been accounted for these specialists, albeit a few patients whined about weariness, unfortunate hunger, unfavourably susceptible responses, edema, skin rash, and neutropenia.252,266 There are a few current clinical preliminaries of HGF/c-MET-designated specialists with regards to CRC treatment (Table 5).

Rather than obstructing HGF actuation, killing HGF to block its capacity to tie to receptors to slow down entire pathway gives off an impression of being more commonsense. A couple of monoclonal antibodies have been combined and presented in a few clinical preliminaries. Rilotumumab, a refined IgG monoclonal neutralizer, has been explored in stage I and II preliminaries. In those patients with gastric or gastroesophageal disease, a drawn out middle PFS (6.8 versus 4.4 months; HR = 0.46, 95% certainty span (CI): 0.25-0.85) and operating system (10.6 versus 5.7 months; HR = 0.46, 95% CI: 0.24-0.87) were accomplished in patients with MET overexpression utilizing rilotumumab in addition to Cover contrasted and those in the fake treatment in addition to Cover arm.297 Further stage III examinations (RILOMET-1 and RILOMET-2)261,298 in patients with untreated or high level stage gastric or gastroesophageal malignant growth were stopped early due to a fast expansion in sickness related passings. These preliminaries featured the significance of definition. Current preliminaries usually apply strategies, for example, IHC or FISH to decide the presence of MET overexpression, and a further scoring framework as indicated by the level of growth cells with high staining power is utilized to separate MET-positive/high and MET-negative/low patients, albeit the measures contrast by little degrees.

For patients with CRC, a randomized stage Ib/II trial299 concerning rilotumumab or ganitumab versus panitumumab in patients with KRAS-wild-type metastatic CRC showed no huge advantage with the joined utilization of rilotumumab and panitumumab regarding middle operating system (13.8 versus 13.7 months, p = 0.71) in patients with MET-high illness contrasted and MET-low sickness.

Ficlatuzumab is a refined IgG monoclonal neutralizer that has been explored in a stage I preliminary for cutting edge strong growths and liver metastases.300 TAK-701, one more acculturated enemy of HGF monoclonal neutralizer, was joined with gefitinib to assist with conquering EGFR obstruction in cellular breakdown in the lungs and is likewise going through a stage I trial.301,302,303

MET adversaries

Specialists that contend with HGF for restricting to MET bring about strange dimerization and corruption of MET. Different antibodies have been created, including onartuzumab, DN-30, and ABT-700. Onartuzumab, a murine-determined monoclonal immune response with high explicitness for the MET semaphorin domain,304 has been assessed in a few preliminaries in patients with strong growths, like NSCLC, glioblastoma, gastroesophageal disease, gastric disease, and CRC.305,306,307,308 Worked on middle operating system and PFS were seen in MET-positive cellular breakdown in the lungs patients treated with erlotinib in a stage II preliminary; in any case, no such viability was accounted for in a stage III trial.306 Comparatively, in gastric or gastroesophageal disease, no huge improvement in PFS or operating system was noticed utilizing onartuzumab in addition to mFOLFOX6 versus fake treatment in addition to mFOLFOX6.305 On account of metastatic CRC, no tremendous contrasts were recognized in PFS between MET-positive and MET-negative patients utilizing onartuzumab joined with mFOLFOX6 + bevacizumab or placebo.308

There are a couple of novel MET antibodies that capability promisingly in malignant growth control yet need supporting information in CRC. The neutralizer DN-30 ties to the IPT (Ig-like, plexins, record factors) space of MET and shows a promising skill to repress the multiplication of MET-positive gastric disease and metastatic melanoma in vitro and in vivo.309 ABT-700 is a refined immune response that could prompt gastric and liver growth relapse in preclinical malignant growth models with MET enhancement and passed a stage I preliminary in a few strong growths with good wellbeing and tolerability.310,311,312 Emibetuzumab, an acculturated counter acting agent focusing on MET, has been utilized in stage I and II preliminaries for NSCLC and gastric cancer.313,314,315,316 Other enemy of MET specialists, for example, ABBV-399, YYB-101, and ARGX-111, are either going through or simply past stage I preliminaries for a scope of strong cancers.

Cooperation with the stomach micro biota

The stomach microbiota is firmly connected with carcinogenesis and growth movement of novel methodologies for CRC screening and reconnaissance may be accomplished through single or various microbial markers. Modification of and mediation in the microbiome could likewise add to CRC treatment and further help with foreseeing and observing treatment reaction and unfavorable occasions. Albeit most discoveries have been primer and anticipate clinical approval, the stomach microbiota addresses one of most encouraging methodologies for personalized CRC treatment.

Current chemotherapy for CRC has been displayed to possibly be intervened by the stomach microbiota, which could answer cytotoxic specialists by means of modifications of their variety, area, and metabolism.466,468,469,470 Explicit kinds of creatures in the stomach microbiota have been found to assume a crucial part in protection from 5-FU and Bull treatment by interceding autophagy.471 what's more, other stomach occupants could irritate chemotherapy-related unfriendly responses through microbial digestion of chemotherapy specialists, for example, IRI.472 There is restricted proof showing that the stomach microbiota could slow down designated treatment; nonetheless, have microbiome collaborations in trial settings could propose a few hidden hints for the microbial-intervened viability of designated specialists. Bile acids are among the major microbial metabolic items, which are additionally applicable to the inception and movement of CRC.473 The crosstalk between the stomach microbiota and the host gastrointestinal cells is viewed as interceded by the movement of essential optional bile corrosive change, which fundamentally controls the development of colon epithelial cells by means of EGFR and atomic farnesoid X receptor signaling.474 Subsequently, more examination is expected to affirm that microbial intercessions, like the utilization of probiotics, could decrease digestive irritation through EGFR guideline. No additional proof has been introduced expressing that EGFR-designated treatment may be impeded by the stomach microbiota. Comparable ends can be drawn for hostile to VEGF treatment, which might be significantly more connected with the stomach microbiota. An angiogenesis-interceded capability for the stomach microbiota was accounted for already, by which the malignant growth microenvironment was framed and shaped.475,476 Probiotics could assist with controlling nearby irritation by down regulating the VEGF/VEGFR pathway in the liver and gastrointestinal cells.477,478 Anti-microbial use, which could decisively lessen stomach microbial variety and thickness, was viewed as connected with unfortunate endurance in patients with metastatic CRC who had gotten bevacizumab therapy.479 In any case, the impact of the microbiota on enemy of VEGF specialists is as yet a question of discussion due to the disputable detailed results480,481 in renal cell disease based examinations expressing a muddled job of anti-infection agents in VEGF-bar treatment.

Curiously, the stomach microbiota ended up being a key component for resistant designated spot barricade and impacted reactions and unfavorable reactions.482,483,484,485,486 A few kinds of microorganisms were connected with the medication response,487,488,489,490,491,492 and further examinations showed that colonization by a mix of 11 types of microscopic organisms in microbe free mice could have improved the viability of safe designated spot modulators, to some extent on the grounds that the new bacterial contamination prompted more grounded safe defensive penetration and reaction from CD8+ Lymphocytes, as well as expanded quantities of CD4+ Lymphocytes and CD103+/MHC class Ia-communicating dendritic cells.493 Anti-toxin openness was related with diminished clinical movement because of immunotherapy with a diminished PFS and operating system in NSCLC (PFS: 1.9 versus 3.8 months, HR = 1.5, p = 0.03; operating system: 7.9 versus 24.6 months, HR = 4.4, p < 0.01) and renal malignant growth (PFS: 1.9 versus 7.4 months, HR = 3.1, p < 0.01; operating system: 17.3 versus 30.6 months, HR = 3.5, p = 0.03),489 discoveries that have been repeated by ongoing investigations that showed an emphatically diminished immunotherapeutic advantage (2 versus 26 months, HR = 7.4) whenever anti-microbial were given for a few malignant growth types.494,495 Comparatively, the viability of a PD-1 inhibitor in melanoma patients corresponded with the stomach microbiota, and reconstitution of the microbiota from PD-1 treatment answering patients could bring about an upgraded White blood cell reaction and further developed PD-1-hindering impact, while transplantations from nonresponding patients had a negative outcome.490,491,492 Further metagenomics examination recognized Akkermansia muciniphila as the key microorganisms that improves PD-1 bar, however this impact may be overwhelmed by the organization of antibiotics.496,497 likewise, the stomach microbiota could foresee immunotherapy-related colitis in light of the fact that enhanced degrees of Firmicutes demonstrated a more successive event of ipilimumab-prompted colitis.488 Right now, a couple of preliminaries are in progress researching whether immunotherapy can be changed by waste microbiota transplantation (NCT04130763, NCT04116775, and NCT03341143). Be that as it may, much still needs to be found out about the stomach microbiota in safe reaction guideline, and explaining the fundamental component requires further examination. Besides, an absence of powerful strategies to exactly control the overflow or constitution of explicit strains or gatherings of the stomach microbiota limits the ongoing open doors for mediation.

Different pathways

The advancement of new designated specialists in light of pathways other than recently realized ones seems, by all accounts, to be somewhat sluggish. A couple of clinical preliminaries concerning drugs focused on targets like IGF-1R, Wnt, Indent, Hedgehog, human demise receptor 5 and TGF-β have been started, yet no appealing outcomes have arisen up until this point. For instance, the γ-secretase inhibitor RO4929097 in Score bar treatment and the Hedgehog pathway inhibitor vismodegib showed little impact in stage II trials.498,499 The restricted advancement of hostile to TGF-β and hostile to Wnt treatment against CRC has likewise been reviewed.500,501 Specialists, for example, COX-2 inhibitors were viewed as accommodating in CRC anticipation regarding hindrance; in any case, the improvement of different specialists that could upgrade chemotherapy responsiveness, yet direct CRC-control-designated drugs with high fondness to single targets, actually lingers behind. The presence of hybrid between these pathways has additionally made bar treatment wasteful, and different obstructions, for example, troubles in choosing patients who will answer well, recognizing result screen markers, and proficiently hindering explicit targets, have showed up; nonetheless, these poor person stopped examinations concerning novel specialists. Table 8 sums up those specialists under clinical examination for different targets.

www.ingramcontent.com/pod-product-compliance
Lightning Source LLC
Chambersburg PA
CBHW070750250726
48662CB00004B/1733